Hi! My name is Tommy
and I am 6 years old.

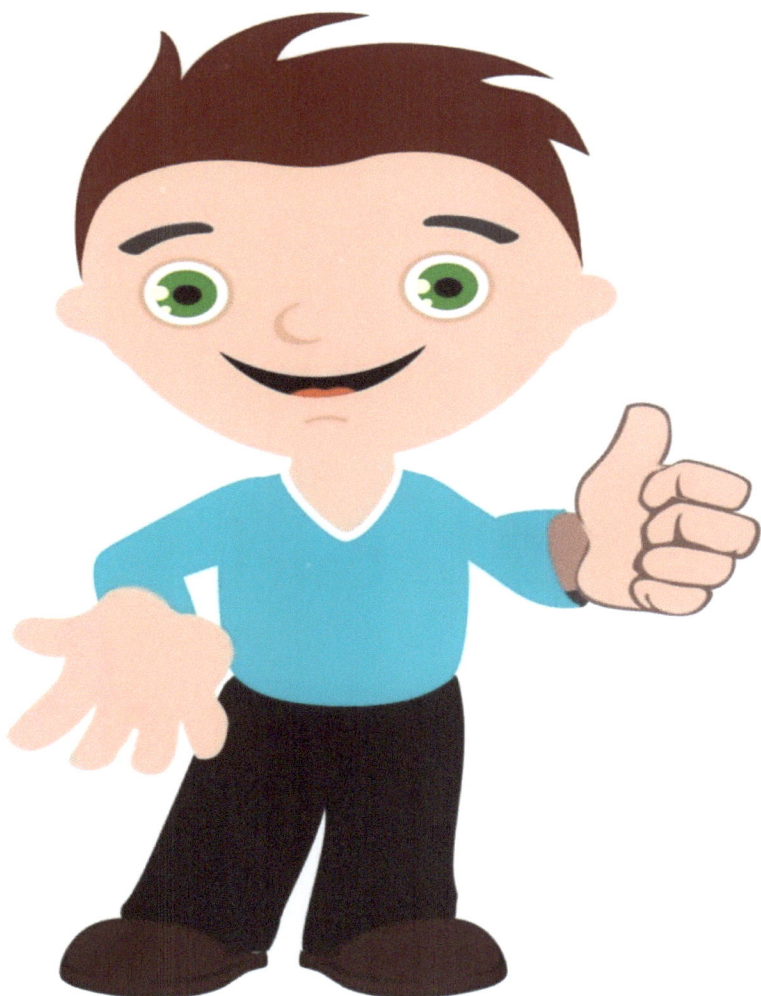

I live with my Mommy, Daddy, and our dog Camio.

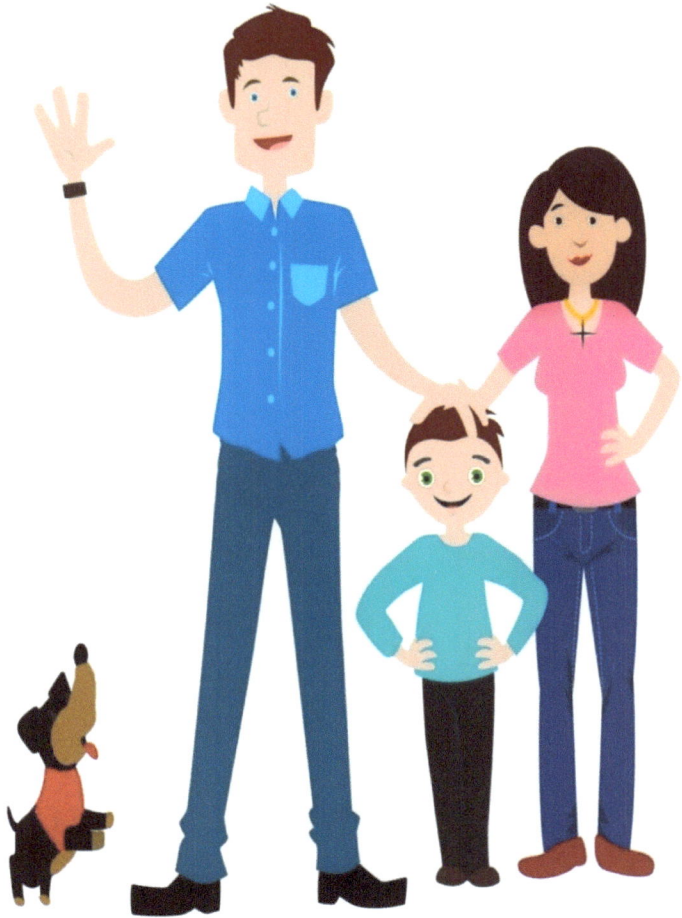

I go to Kindergarten and have the best friends in my class!

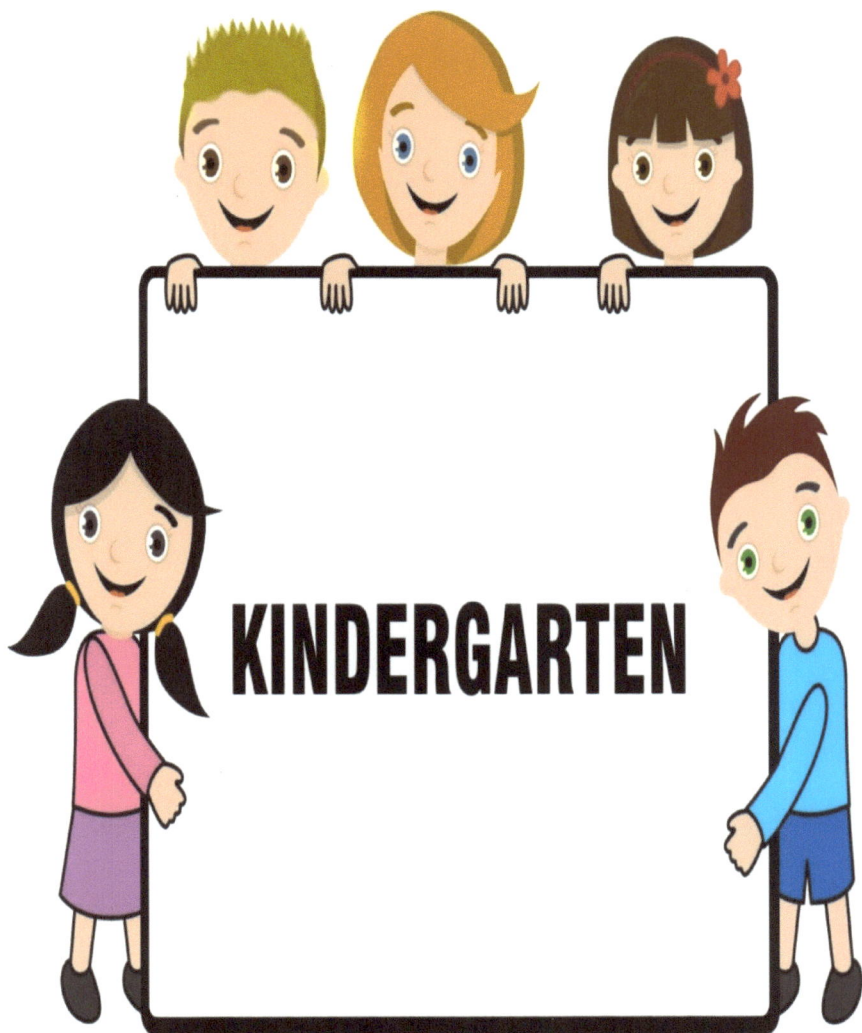

KINDERGARTEN

I play baseball, soccer, and take karate lessons.

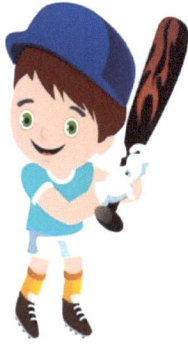

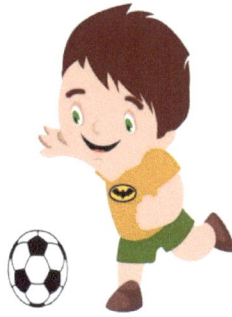

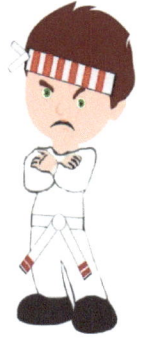

Sometimes I fall and hurt myself...doesn't everybody?

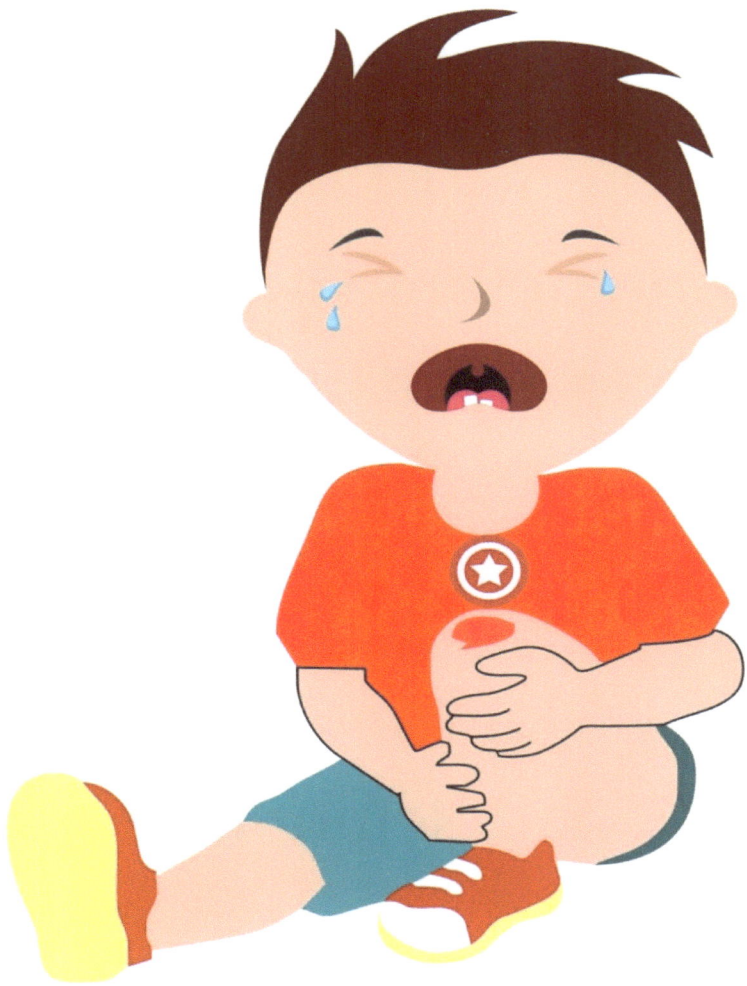

But when *I* get hurt, sometimes I need more than just a band-aid.

That is because when I was born, the doctors told my Mom and Dad that I had Hemophilia.

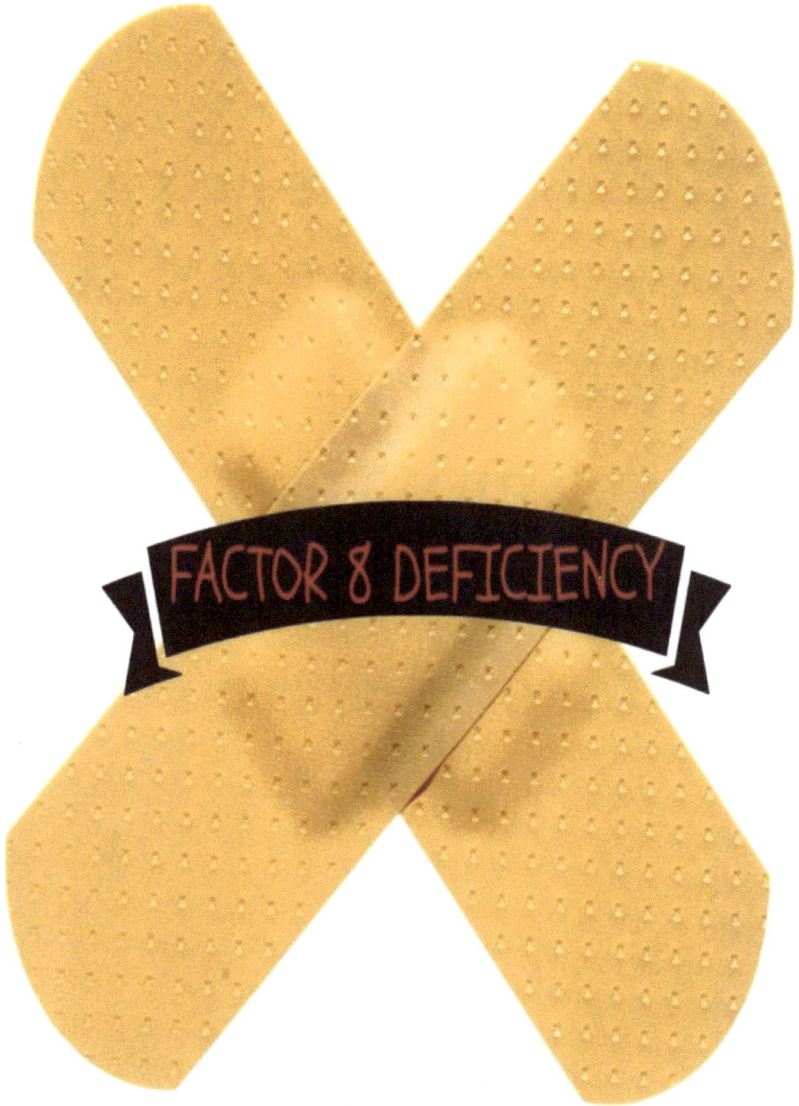

FACTOR 8 DEFICIENCY

Hemophilia is just a big word that means that my blood doesn't clot very well on its own. I get medication to help my blood form clots in case of an injury.

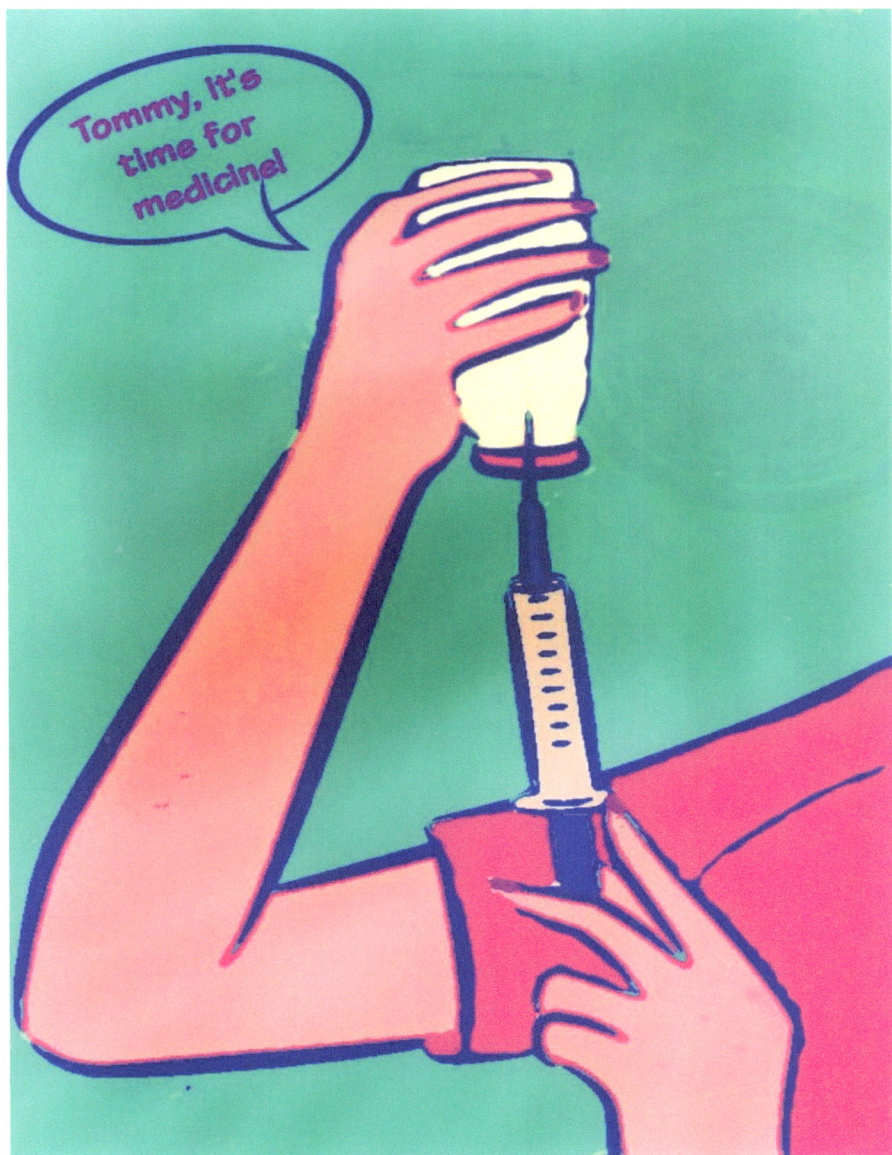

Sometimes I get mad when it's time for medicine because I just want to keep playing.

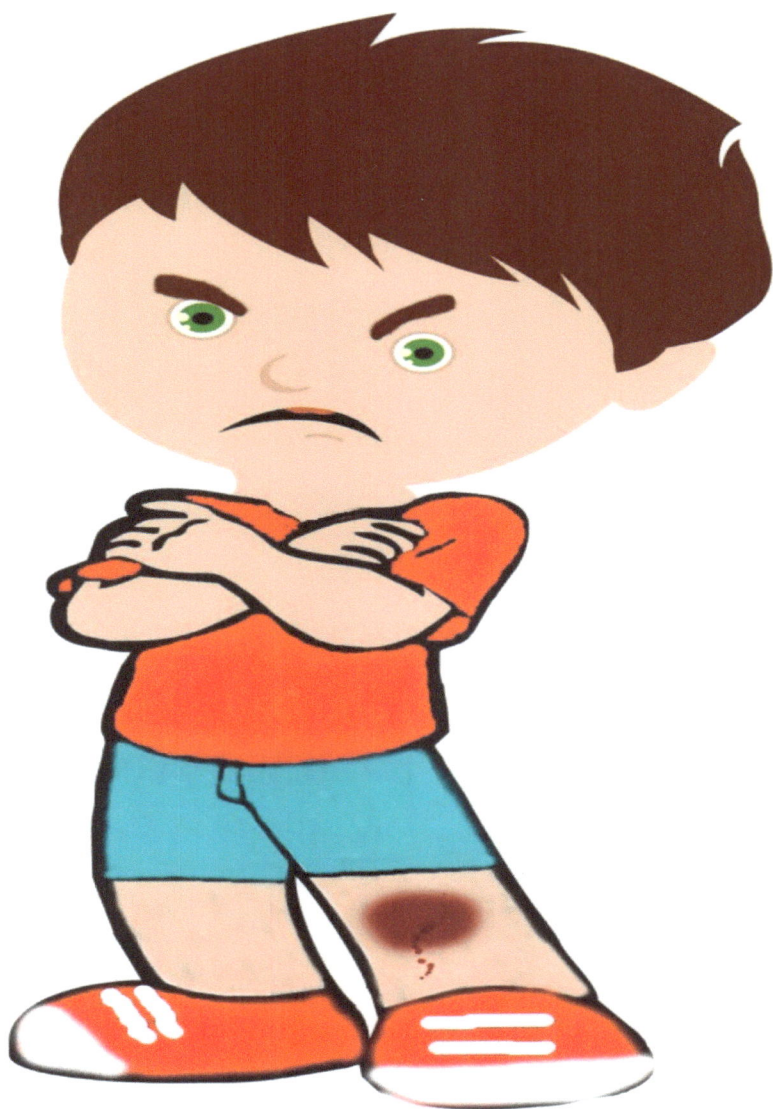

But now that I am 6 years old, Mom and Dad let me help them set up the supplies for medicine time. I can clean my vein with an alcohol wipe and then spray Freeze Spray over my vein so that I can't feel the needle when it goes in. I have learned that if I sit as still as a statue, the needle part is over very quickly and it doesn't even hurt most of the time either! Mom and Dad even let me push the medicine through the syringe into my vein and then let me remove the needle! That makes me feel happy and important to help.

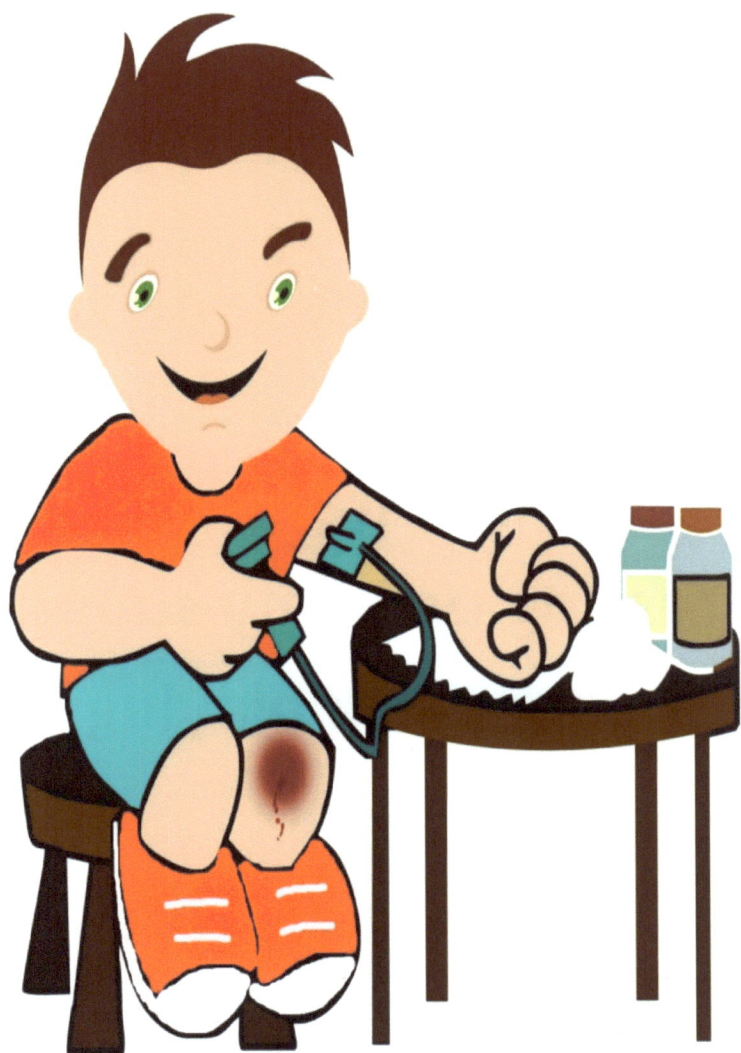

Once medicine time is over, I can go right back to doing my favorite things like dressing up in my superhero costumes and playing video games!

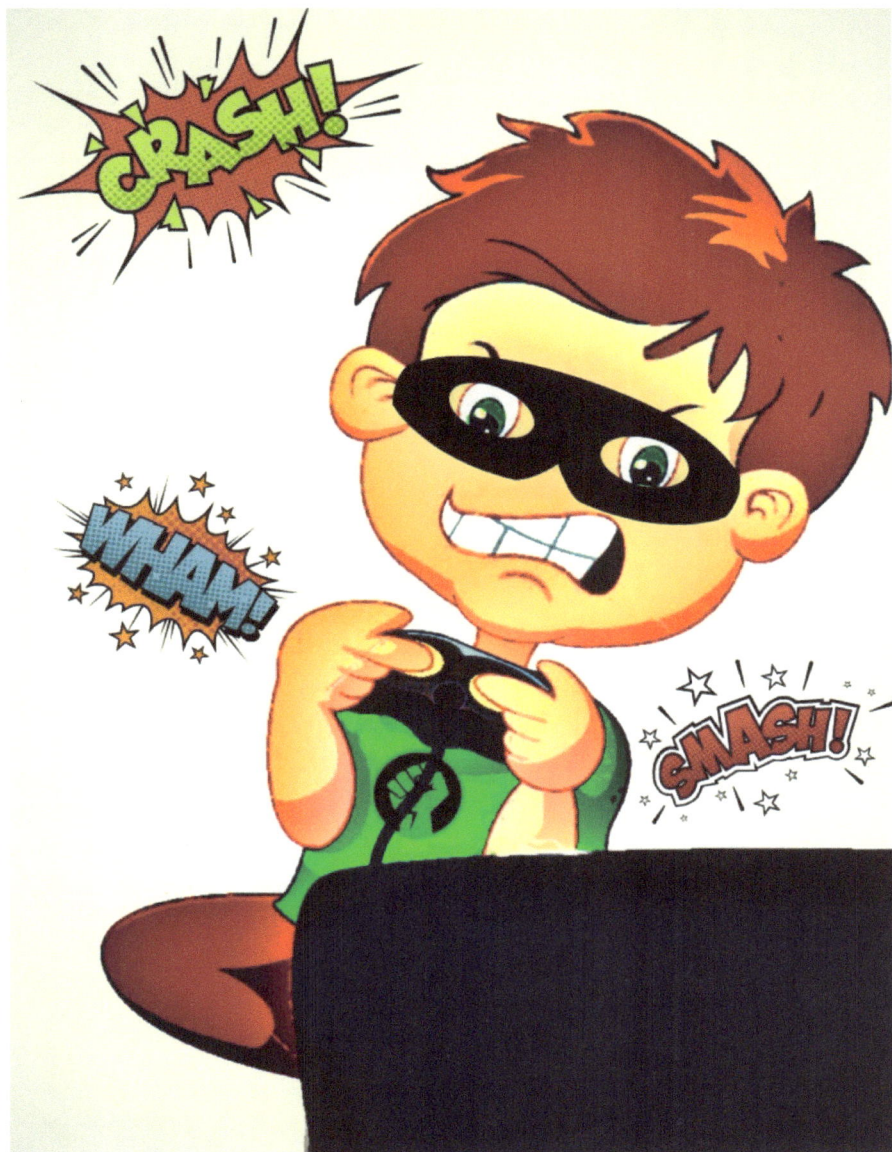

Having Hemophilia isn't so bad at all! I can still do everything I want to do as long as I am careful and tell Mom and Dad anytime I hurt myself. Mom and Dad tell me that I can be whatever I want to be when I grow up too. I think I want to be a superhero. After all, Mommy and Daddy always say I am their hero!

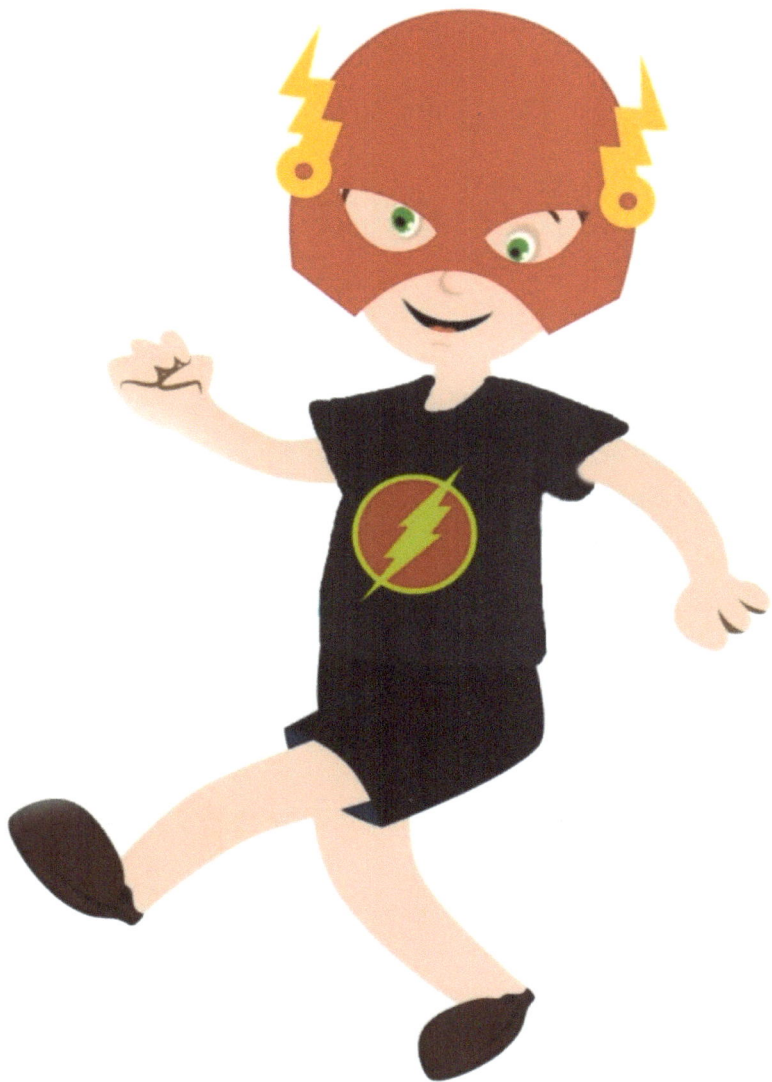

About Tommy

Tommy is a 6 year old who was diagnosed at 5 days old with Severe Hemophilia type A. His body produces less than 1% of an essential clotting protein called Factor VIII. At age 2, Tommy developed an inhibitor to the Factor VIII medication. He underwent surgery to have a port installed in his chest in order to begin Immune Tolerance to rid his body of this inhibitor. After many daily infusions of Factor VIII, he was declared inhibitor free and was reverted back to every other day infusions of Factor VIII. Sadly, the inhibitor returned once again and everyday infusions began as well. At the time of this writing,

Tommy is on the second round of Immune Tolerance and doing well. The inhibitor has measured at an extremely low number for the past two months and we look forward to reverting back to our "normal" life of every other day infusions in the near future.

www.ingramcontent.com/pod-product-compliance
Lightning Source LLC
Chambersburg PA
CBHW041224270326
41933CB00001B/42